National Health
and Nutrition
Examination Survey

BALANCE
PROCEDURES
MANUAL

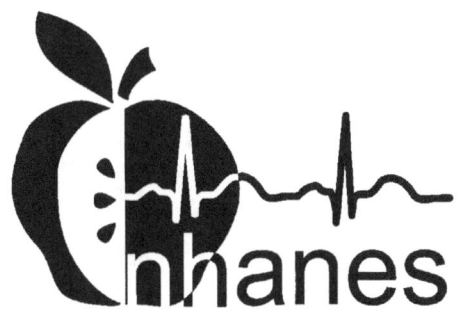

(Revised January 2003)

TABLE OF CONTENTS

TABLE OF CONTENTS (Continued)

List of Exhibits

1. INTRODUCTION TO THE BALANCE COMPONENT

1.1   Background

The ability to maintain balance is essential to nearly all activities associated with daily living. The balance system enables us to sense where we are in space and to maintain our posture and equilibrium while we are still and while we are in movement. We often do not consider balance as a "sense" in the same way that we think of seeing, hearing, tasting, smelling, and so on, because balance is usually an automatic, unconscious process. However, impairment of the balance system can be a major disabling condition for those who are affected.

The control of balance requires the integration of information from multiple sensory and motor systems by the central nervous system (CNS). Balance receptors in the inner ear (the vestibular system) provide information to the CNS about head and body movements. The eyes (visual system) provide input regarding the body's orientation within the environment and about motion within the environment. The position and motion sensors of the muscles and joints, and the touch receptors of the extremities (proprioceptive system) send signals regarding bodily position, particularly in relation to the support surface. The CNS integrates all this data, determines the body's spatial orientation, and sends appropriate neural messages to the motor system to activate movements that will maintain equilibrium.

Because the balance system is so complex, it can be impaired by a large number of disease processes affecting any of the multiple sensory inputs, neural processing centers, or motor outputs. These include (but are not limited to) infections of the inner ear, head injury, drug or environmental toxicity, cerebrovascular insults, degenerative changes due to aging or illness, and autoimmune reactions. Balance disorders can result in a wide variety of symptoms, ranging from a generalized feeling of disorientation and disequilibrium to acute vertigo (i.e., the sensation of motion, particularly spinning of the body or the environment). Because balance is normally an unconscious process, patients often have difficulty articulating their symptoms; and physicians can have difficulty determining the exact cause of the problem.

Impairments of balance are common and debilitating conditions. People with chronic balance disorders are significantly disabled in many day-to-day functions, particularly those that require stabilizing the body during weight-shifting, bending, or rapid head motion. Examples of such tasks include getting in and out of bed, taking a bath or shower, climbing stairs, and reaching for objects in high or low cabinets. Changes in body posture that require shifting one's weight or moving the head are particularly problematic, and can induce vertigo. In addition, those who have balance impairments have more difficulty than normal individuals doing tasks that involve spatial perception and movement, and often report bumping into walls, walking off a sidewalk, or veering into another lane while driving (Cohen 1992, Cohen et al., 1995). Balance disorders restrict an individual's normal motor activities, thereby limiting one's sense of independence and adversely affecting the quality of life.

The prevalence of balance disorders in the overall population of the United States is unknown. It is estimated that at least half of the overall population of the United States are affected by a balance or vestibular disorder sometime during life. Several groups are particularly at risk. The National Institute on Deafness and Other Communication Disorders (NIDCD) estimates that up to two-thirds of children with acquired deafness have severe vestibular deficits (NIDCD, 1995). In addition, individuals who have sustained head injuries are likely to suffer from problems with balance and dizziness (NIDCD, 1995). Healthy individuals who are exposed to unusual motion and gravity environments, such as divers, high-speed pilots, and astronauts, are another affected group (NIDCD, 1989).

The elderly, in particular, have a higher risk of balance impairments due to the several alterations in function associated with aging. The NIDCD (1995) estimates that 12.5 million Americans over the age of 65 have dizziness or balance problems that significantly interfere with their lives. Data from the National Ambulatory Medical Care Survey, conducted by the National Center for Health Statistics (NCHS), indicated that disequilibrium was one of the two most common diagnoses among short-stay hospital admissions for individuals over the age of 65. It also found that dizziness was the most common complaint presented to primary care physicians among patients 75 years of age and older (Cypress, 1981). There is evidence that with aging, the control of balance is increasingly dependent on visual and proprioceptive cues, making older individuals more vulnerable to falls when those orientation cues are degraded (Peterka and Black, 1990). Over one-half of accidental deaths among the elderly are the result of balance-related falls (NIDCD, 1989).

Timed tests of balance during stance and locomotion were administered to persons 60 years of age and older in NHANES III. Their ability to stand heel-to-toe for a specified period of time, and the length of time required to walk a specified distance were evaluated. While this data provides rough estimates as to the prevalence of balance trouble among older adults, it does not provide any data on the relative severity of the disorder nor any clue as to a probable site of lesion.

The balance component of NHANES is designed to assess the prevalence of balance disorders among adults aged 40 years and older. Specifically, the goals of the NHANES balance component are:

■   To determine the prevalence of balance deficits among adults aged 40 years and older;

■   To identify risk factors that predispose individuals to balance disorders, so that preventive interventions may be established; and

■   To help health planners in the Federal, state, local, and private sectors to predict the impact of the "baby boomer" generation on the health care resources and services needed in the future as the population ages.

The examination that will be used in the NHANES balance component is called the Romberg Test of Standing Balance on Firm and Compliant Support Surfaces. It is a proven and standardized protocol that is commonly used as a screening instrument in balance assessment in both clinical and research settings. It is designed to identify deficits in standing balance; however, it is not designed to diagnose the cause of a particular balance problem.

The Romberg Test is quick and simple to administer. Standardized procedures have been developed for conducting and scoring the test. You will receive extensive training to ensure that you understand and can implement all aspects of the protocol. It is critical that you follow the procedures exactly, so that data on each examinee is collected in a uniform manner. If you are ever uncertain about anything regarding the procedure or a particular examinee, ask your supervisor.

Before learning the protocol for the NHANES balance component, it is important to understand some basic information about the balance system and its disorders. This knowledge will be helpful in your implementation of the protocol.

1.2   Basic Anatomy of the Balance System

The body's ability to maintain balance depends on (1) inputs from three body systems (the vestibular, visual, and proprioceptive systems), (2) integration of these inputs by the CNS, and (3) appropriate responses to the integrated signal by the body's musculoskeletal system.

The primary organs of balance, the vestibular sensors, are located within the inner ear. Attached to the cochlea (the snail-shaped organ that converts sound into neural signals) are three semicircular canals. The canals are aligned to form a coordinate system, so that one canal lies in each plane (see figure below). The semicircular canals are encased in the temporal bone of the skull, and are filled with fluid. At the base of each canal is an enlarged area called the ampulla, which contains a receptor organ, the cupulla, containing tiny hair cells that project into the gelatinous composition of the cupulla. At the base of these hair cells are fibers from the vestibular branch of the eighth cranial nerve (CNVIII), which carries their sensory input to the CNS.

Exhibit 1-1. Cochlea and semicircular canals (right and left)

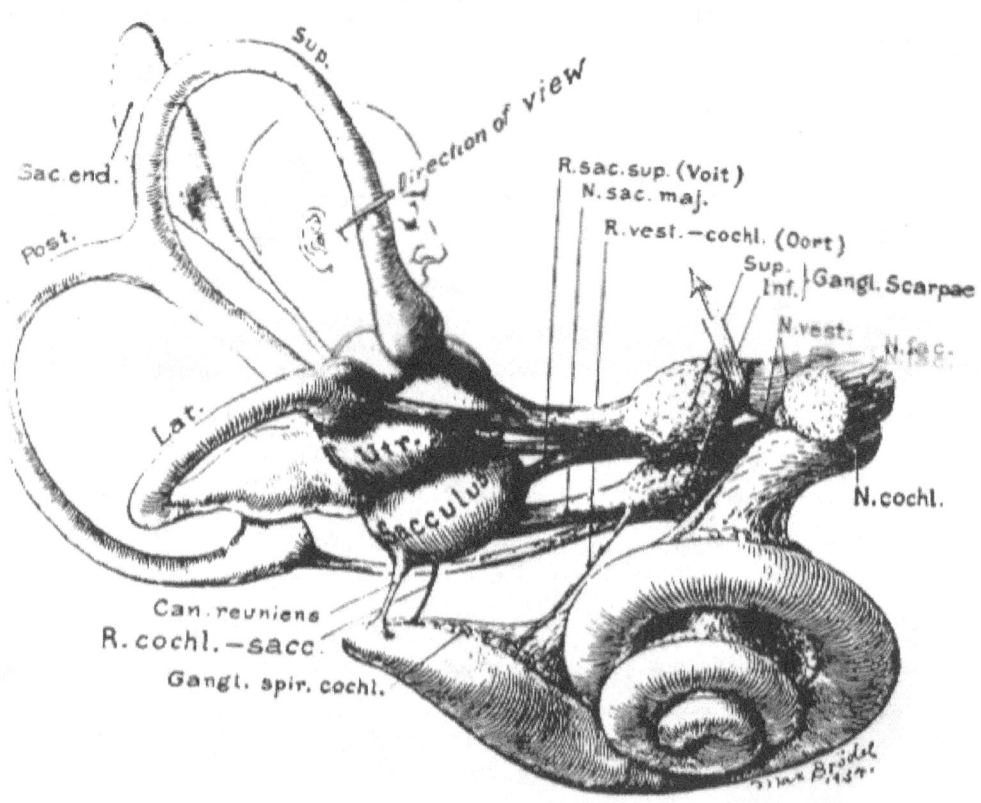

The fluid in the semicircular canals moves in response to pivoting movements of the head, such as turning, tilting, or bending. The movement of the fluid causes the hair cells in the ampullae to bend, changing the neural signals which are sent to the brain. The fluid in each ear moves in opposite directions, so that hair cells in the ampullae are also bent in opposite directions. For example, if you turn your head to the right, the fluid in your right horizontal semicircular canal moves in a direction which causes the vestibular sensor on that side to send additional neural impulses to the brain. At the same time, the hair cells of corresponding vestibular sensor on the left are bent in the other direction, causing fewer impulses to be sent. The brain interprets this difference in neural signals as head movement.

Between the cochlea and the semicircular canals is a space in the temporal bone called the vestibule. In this space, which is also fluid-filled, lie two organs, the utricle and saccule, which respond to linear (to-and-fro) motion of the head and to the force, or pull, of gravity. The utricle and saccule contain hair cells imbedded in a gelatinous covering (membrane) that contains tiny crystals, called otoconia. The otoconia press against the hair cells with a pressure proportionate to the head motion and to the pull of gravity. This information is sent to the brain to enable us to maintain our spatial orientation and balance.

Information from the visual and proprioceptive systems is sent to the brain and interpreted in conjunction with the signals from the vestibular system. The brain then sends out appropriate neural impulses that stimulate reflexive actions in the musculoskeletal system to cause the body to react as necessary to maintain balance.

Sometimes the brain must decide between conflicting inputs. For example, when you suddenly stop spinning, the fluid in your semi-circular canals continues to flow for a few seconds, which tells the brain that you are still moving. However, the input from your visual system tells the brain that you are not. On the other hand, when you are waiting at a stop light and the car next to you pulls slightly forward, your visual system senses that you are rolling backward. However, your vestibular system indicates that you are still at rest. Such sensory conflicts can result in disorientation and motion sickness.

1.3   Disorders of Balance

Because of the complexity of the balance system and the number of sensory and motor mechanisms that contribute toward it, there are many disorders that can disrupt normal balance function. However, even if a disorder cannot be treated medically or surgically, rehabilitation therapy can sometimes be effective in training the other contributory systems to compensate for the impaired system.

Peripheral vestibular disorders are caused by damage to the inner ear balance receptors and/or the nerve (CNVIII) that connects to the receptor organs. Damage can result from infection, head injury, toxicity, or other causes, and can be unilateral (one-sided) or bilateral (two-sided). Unilateral disorders are more common, and often result in a primary symptom of vertigo (a sensation of movement, usually spinning, which results from an imbalance in the neural signals being sent to the brain). Examples of peripheral vestibular disorders include Meniere's disease (an idiopathic fluctuation in ear fluids), perilymphatic fistula (a leak of the fluid-filled inner ear), and labyrinthitis (an inner ear infection).

Central vestibular disorders are caused by damage to the central nervous system areas that integrate balance information. This type of damage can result from space-occupying lesions, such as tumors or aneurysms in the brain stem, or from degenerative brain disorders, such as multiple sclerosis or stroke. Central disorders can result in vertigo or more generalized symptoms such as lightheadedness, dizziness, unsteadiness, or ataxia (loss of muscle coordination).

Damage to the visual and/or musculoskeletal system can also result in balance impairment. Systemic disorders such as metabolic abnormalities, autoimmune disease, and psychogenic disturbances (e.g. anxiety disorders) are other potential etiologies of disordered balance.

References

Cohen, H. (1992). Vestibular rehabilitation reduces functional disability. *Arch Otolaryngol Head Neck Surg*, 107:638-643.

Cohen H., Ewell, L.R., and Jenkins, H.A. (1995). Disability in Meniere's Disease. *Arch Otolaryngol Head Neck Surg*, 121:29-33.

Cypress, BK. (1981). *Patients' Reasons for Visiting Physicians: National Medical Ambulatory Care Survey: United States, 1977-1978.* National Center for Health Statistics, PHS Publication No. 82-1717, Hyattsville, Maryland.

NIDCD. (1989). *A Report of the Task Force on the National Strategic Research Plan.* National Institutes of Health, Bethesda, Maryland.

NIDCD. (1995). *National Strategic Plan: Balance and Balance Disorders.* National Institute on Deafness and Other Communication Disorders, National Institutes of Health, NIH Publication No. 96-3217, Bethesda, Maryland.

Peterka, R.J. and Black, F.O. (1990). Age-related changes in human posture control: Sensory organization tests. *J Vest Res*, 1: 73-85.

2. EQUIPMENT AND SUPPLIES

2.1   Description of Exam Room in MEC

The balance examination will be conducted in the shared balance and specimen collection room, located in Trailer #1 of the Mobile Examination Center (MEC). The room has been specially outfitted to ensure the accuracy of the exam results and the safety of examinees throughout the balance test. The room is carpeted and has few visual or auditory distractions, except for the visual target located on the door for fixation during eyes-open testing.

The work area for the health technologist consists of a built-in desk and computer station. There are shelves located below the computer station, on which equipment specific to the balance exam *will be stored* when the room is used for specimen collection and during transit from one stand to another.

2.2   Description of Equipment and Supplies

The following equipment has been supplied for the balance component of NHANES:

■   Sammons Preston velcro walking belt in three sizes (small, medium, and large). This is a safety gait belt with three handles (grab loops), which will enable the technician to steady the examinee if he or she begins to lose balance during the exam. The belt comes in three sizes (S, M, L) based on waist measurement.

■   Stopwatch. The stopwatch will be used to time each test condition.

■   Sunmate medium density foam pad (16" x 18" x 3") and washable lycra cover. The foam pad provides the compliant support surface for Conditions 3 and 4 of the balance protocol. The cover is a 4-way stretch lycra that fits snugly over the foam pad like a pillowcase with a zipper; the cover is incontinent proof and can be machine-washed for hygienic purposes.

An inventory of the balance equipment and supplies will be conducted at the beginning and end of each stand.

3. BALANCE COMPONENT PROTOCOL

3.1   Eligibility Criteria

The balance examination will be conducted on examinees ages 40 years and older.

There are five exclusionary criteria that preclude an examinee from participating in the balance exam:

1.   Inability to stand unassisted;

2.   Prosthetic device below the waist;

3.   Weight exceeding 275 lbs.;

4.   Waist circumference either too small or too large to accommodate proper fitting of any standard sized safety gait belt; and

5.   Current symptoms of dizziness or lightheadedness.

The waist circumference will be determined when the safety belt is put on. Other exclusions will be identified through a brief series of questions asked of the examinee immediately prior to the balance exam to verify their eligibility (see page 3-2).

3.2   Pre-examination Procedures

3.2.1   Preliminary Procedures

Take out the stopwatch, foam pad, and safety belts if these have been put away due to use of the room for specimen collection. The login screen appears when the coordinator assigns an SP to the exam component. Type in your password and click OK.

Each participant will wear an identification bracelet with the participant's identification number barcoded on it. The technician will enter the barcode number into the ISIS system by "reading" the bar code with a wand. ISIS will automatically pull up the identification screen for that examinee. Verify that the SP information is correct. Click OK to continue.

3.2.2   Pre-exam Questions

Before beginning the balance exam, the study participant will be asked a series of questions to identify any conditions that might preclude the person from participating in the test. Screen 1 of the Balance Exam subsystem will prompt you to ask the following questions (see Exhibit 3-1). Answers to the final four questions may preclude the person from the test for safety reasons.

Exhibit 3-1. Exclusion/Safety Questions

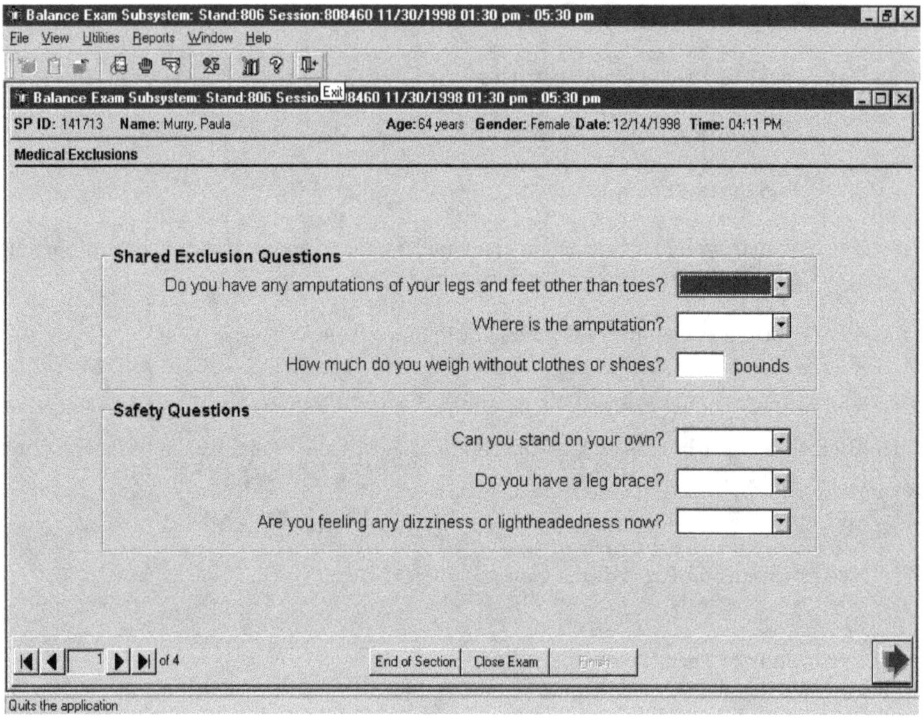

ISIS will default to one answer in each of the questions (bolded below), with the exception of the question on weight. The questions on amputations and weight are questions that are shared with other MEC component exams. Therefore, if a person has provided their weight to another component exam, ISIS will show that weight in the response space for the question in this component.

To complete this section, click on the appropriate response or follow the instructions below.

1.   DO YOU HAVE ANY AMPUTATIONS OF YOUR LEGS AND FEET OTHER THAN TOES?

         YES   **NO**

2.   WHERE IS THE AMPUTATION?

This question provides a drop-down menu of responses. Click on the down-arrow and then one of the three choices.

3.   HOW MUCH DO YOU WEIGH WITHOUT CLOTHES OR SHOES?

A space is provided for you to enter the weight in pounds. If the response is over 275 pounds, a message box (see Exhibit 3-2) will appear on the screen informing you that the SP is excluded from the exam for safety reasons.

Exhibit 3-2. SP exclusion message

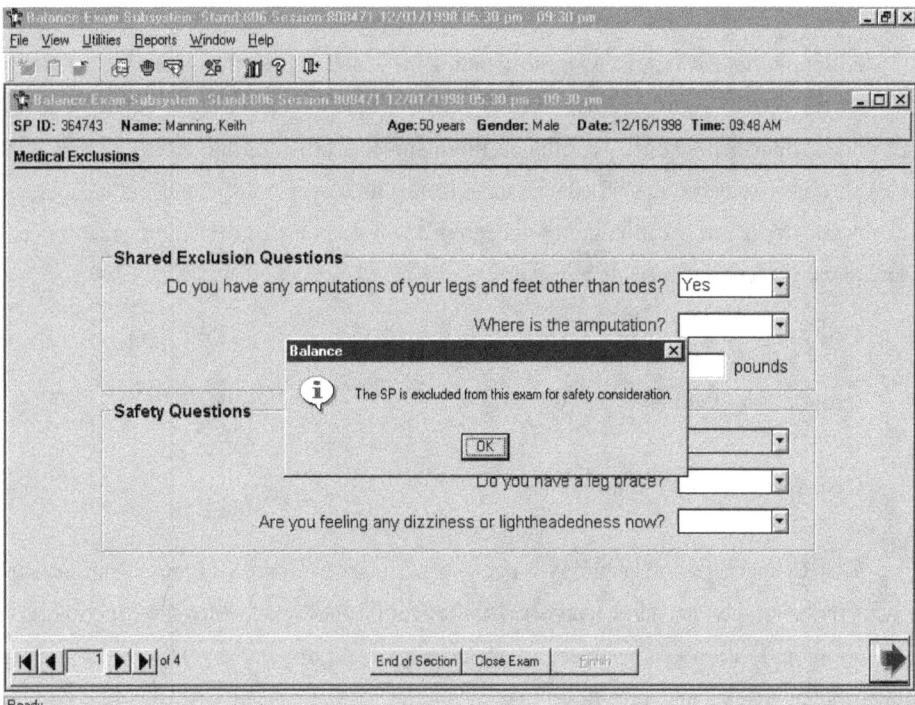

4.   CAN YOU STAND ON YOUR OWN?

YES   NO

"On your own" means without assistance from another person; without use of a device, such as a cane, walker, or leg brace; and without relying on support from a wall, furniture, etc. If the study participant cannot stand unassisted, he cannot undergo the balance exam. A message box (See Exhibit 3.2) will appear on the screen, informing you that the SP is excluded from the exam for safety reasons.

5.   DO YOU HAVE A LEG BRACE?

YES   **NO**

A brace refers to any orthotic device below the waist. This does not include extra-depth or orthopedic shoes or orthotic inserts in shoes. A positive response precludes the examinee from participating in the exam. Again, the message box will appear on the screen to inform you that the sampled person is excluded from the exam.

6. ARE YOU FEELING ANY DIZZINESS OR LIGHTHEADEDNESS NOW?

YES   **NO**

Examinees who are experiencing these symptoms at the time of the test should not take part in the balance exam. Examinees who report periodic dizziness, or even dizziness earlier in the day, are not excluded if they are not symptomatic at the time of the exam.

A final exclusion is severe visual impairment, which impedes valid testing for Balance Test Conditions 1 and 3. Subjects who because of visual handicap need assistance in finding the testing room should not undergo balance testing. To exclude these subjects from testing, at the bottom of the ISIS "Medical Exclusions" screen click "Close Exam". In the following "Not Done Status" screen, under "Reason", select "Other" at the bottom of the drop-down response menu, then type "severe visual impairment" in the text comment field provided.

3.3   Examination Protocol

3.3.1   Description of the Examination

The Romberg Test of Standing Balance on Firm and Compliant Support Surfaces examines the ability of the examinee to stand unassisted under four conditions, ordered in increasing level of difficulty. Condition 1 allows the subject to make use of all the sensory inputs that contribute to balance—vestibular, visual, and proprioceptive. Condition 2 tests balance when only vestibular and proprioceptive information is available; the subject closes his eyes to eliminate the visual input. In Condition 3, the subject must maintain balance on a foam surface, which reduces the proprioceptive input and leaves only visual and vestibular cues. Finally, in Condition 4, the visual input is again removed and the subject's ability to maintain balance using only his vestibular system is tested.

In the standard Balance Testing protocol, each subject is eligible for an initial test and one re-test in order to pass a specific Test Condition. Within each Test Condition, the protocol for retesting is the same as for the primary examination.

Because each successive Test Condition from 1 to 4 is progressively more difficult than the Condition preceding it, the Balance Testing Component is ended whenever a subject fails to pass a condition.

3.3.2   Preparation of the Examinee

Explain the purpose of the balance examination using the following standard script:

> "This is a series of quick tests to see how well you can maintain your balance under various conditions. Each test simply involves having to stand still for a short length of time. I am not going to do anything "tricky" or purposely try to make you lose your balance. You will just be standing still."

Explain to the examinee that you are going to place a safety belt around his or her waist as a precaution in the event the examinee should feel unsteady at any point during the test. Determine the appropriate size safety belt based on the subject's waist size. It is not necessary to measure the waist; a judgement call will generally be adequate. Wrap the belt around the participant's waist, such that the grab loops are in the front, and secure it snugly (but not tightly) with the Velcro closure. If the subject's waist is either too large or too small for any belt to fit securely, the subject should be excluded from the exam.

Point out that the walls serve as support that will be available to the subject if he or she feels unsteady; and emphasize that you will be within reach at all times to prevent him from falling.

3.3.3   The Four Test Conditions

3.3.3.1   Test Condition 1

Screen number 2 contains the data entry areas for test conditions 1 and 2 (see Exhibit 3-3).

Exhibit 3-3. Exam Conditions 1 and 2

File View Utilities Reports Window Help

Balance: Stand:500 Session:500820 12/22/1999 08:30 am - 12:30 pm

SP ID: 699437   Name: JEFFREYS, THANH   Age: 60 years Gender: Male   Date: 03/06/2000 Time: 02:56 PM

Balance Test1 - Feet Together Firm Support (15 seconds)

Condition 1

Stand in this position with your eyes open, looking at the target for as long as you can or until I ask you to stop.
Please do not talk once the test begins.   "Begin now."

Feet together eyes open:	○ pass	Number of Seconds:	
	○ DNP	Reasons:	
Feet together eyes open:	○ pass	Number of Seconds:	
	○ DNP	Reasons:	

Condition 2

Stand in this position with your eyes closed, facing the target for as long as you can or until I ask you to stop.
First assume this position with your eyes open, and then close your eyes. Please do not talk once the test
begins.   "Begin now."

Feet together eyes closed:	○ pass	Number of Seconds:	
	○ DNP	Reasons:	
Feet together eyes closed:	○ pass	Number of Seconds:	
	○ DNP	Reasons:	

|◀ ◀   2   ▶ ▶| of 4   End of Session   Close Exam   Graph   ▶|

Ready | Not connected to Coordinator | 03:03 PM

Direct the examinee to stand facing the visual target on the door. Stand with your feet together and your arms folded across the waist, holding the elbows with the hands (see illustration below), to demonstrate your meaning. Instruct the examinee using the following standard script:

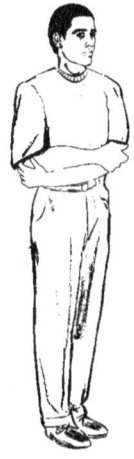

"Stand in this position - with your feet together and your arms and hands at your waist like this. Keep your eyes open and look at the target. Remain in this position for as long as you can or until I ask you to stop. I will let you know when we are ready to begin; and then please do not talk until we are finished with this part of the test. Do you have any questions?"

Proper positioning of the foot is for the SP to place his/her feet together with both heels and great toes touching. In rare instances, if necessary, slight deviations in the spread of feet are acceptable for SPs who for *physical* reasons (such as obesity or leg deformity) are unable to put their feet completely together. An exception *should not* be made to make the exam easier for SPs who cannot place their feet together due to balance trouble.

You must be positioned to assist the subject should they lose their balance. In fact, you should always assume that they will, so that you are alert to helping them. Stand perpendicular to the subject, that is, to their right side, facing them. Keep one hand, your right hand, free to assist the subject. Keep the stopwatch in your left hand. When the examinee has assumed the correct position, say "Ready? Begin." and begin timing. Once the stopwatch has been activated, there should be no talking by anyone in the room.

Do not look at the stopwatch during the test. Instead, mentally count the seconds until the test is finished. For safety and scoring purposes, keep your eyes on the SP at all times, observing them closely throughout the trial. Exact times to failure can be read from the stopwatch after the test is finished. Stop the test after <u>15 seconds,</u> or whenever the subject does something that constitutes a failure (see Scoring Protocol, page 3-11). Stop the watch, and tell the examinee "OK, you may stop now."

Click on the pass or DNP (did not pass) button to record the test result. If the SP failed the condition, you will need to enter the number of seconds that had passed when the failure occurred, plus the reason for the failure. Click on the drop-down menu and click on the appropriate outcome.

If the examinee was able to maintain the stance for 15 seconds, continue with Condition 2.

If the examinee was unable to maintain the stance for 15 seconds, offer to conduct a retrial of the condition by asking, "Can we try that again?" This encourages the SP to do the retrial without sounding optional, or forcing the SP to do a retrial. If necessary, you may allow the subject up to 1 minute to reorient himself between trials. If the examinee agrees to try again, repeat the condition exactly as before. If the examinee does not want to try again, the balance examination should be terminated (see Section 3.6), by clicking on the "Close" button on the navigation bar.

If the examinee was unable to maintain the stance in Condition 1 for 15 seconds, the balance examination should be terminated (see Section 3.6).

3.3.3.2   Test Condition 2

If the SP passes Condition 1, the two trials of Condition 2 become available for data entry.

Direct the examinee to stand facing the visual target on the door. Demonstrate the proper stance again and instruct the examinee using the following standard script:

> "Stand in the same position as before—with your feet together and your arms and hands at your waist like this. This time, however, during the test you will have your eyes closed. When I tell you, close your eyes and remain in this position with your eyes closed for as long as you can or until I ask you to stop. I will let you know when we are ready to begin; and then please do not talk until we are finished with this part of the test. Do you have any questions?"

When both you and the examinee have assumed the correct position, say "Ready? Close your eyes. Begin." and begin the stopwatch. Once the stopwatch is activated, there should be no talking by anyone in the room.

Do not look at the stopwatch during the test. Instead, mentally count the seconds until the test is finished. For safety and scoring purposes, keep your eyes on the SP at all times, observing them closely throughout the trial. Exact times to failure can be read from the stopwatch after the test is finished. Stop the test after 15 seconds, or whenever the subject does something that constitutes a failure (see

Scoring Protocol, page 3-11). Stop the watch, and tell the examinee "OK, you may open your eyes and stop now."

Click on the pass or DNP button to record the result, and to the "number of seconds" and "reason for failure" data as necessary.

If the examinee was able to maintain the stance for 15 seconds, continue with Condition 3.

Advance to Conditions 3 or 4 by clicking on the forward arrow on the navigation bar.

If the examinee was unable to maintain the stance for 15 seconds, offer to conduct a retrial of the condition by asking, "Can we try that again?" This encourages the SP to do the retrial without sounding optional, or forcing the SP to do a retrial. If necessary, you may allow the subject up to 1 minute to reorient himself between trials. If the examinee agrees to try again, repeat the condition exactly as before. If the examinee does not want to try again, the balance examination should be terminated (see Section 3.6), by clicking on the "Close" button on the navigation bar. Advance to Conditions 3 and 4 by clicking on the forward arrow on the navigation bar.

3.3.3.3   Test Condition 3

Test Conditions 3 and 4 are found on page 3 of the application (see Exhibit 3-4).

Exhibit 3-4. Exam Conditions 3 and 4

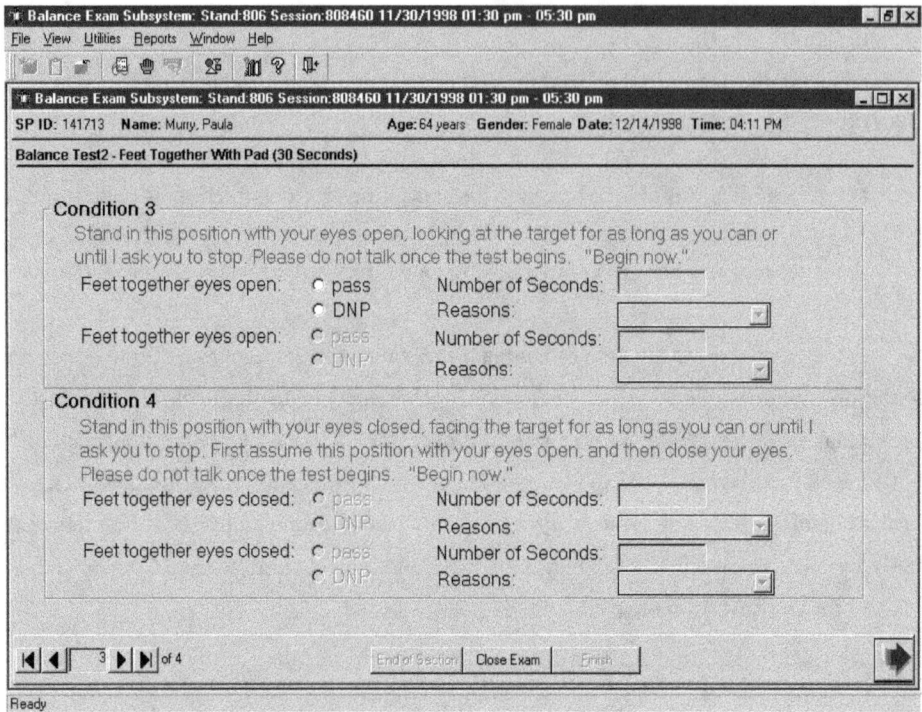

Place the foam pad on the floor where the examinee will stand for the test. Again demonstrating the proper stance *(but without standing on the foam yourself)*, instruct the examinee using the following standard script:

"This test will be much like the first test, except you will be standing on the foam. Stand in the same position—with your feet together and your arms and hands at your waist like this. Keep your eyes open and look at the target. Remain in this position for as long as you can or until I ask you to stop. I will let you know when we are ready to begin; and then please do not talk until we are finished with this part of the test. Do you have any questions?"

Direct the examinee to step onto the center of the foam pad, facing the visual target on the door. When both you and the examinee have assumed the correct position, say "Ready? Start." and begin the stopwatch. Once the watch is activated, there should be no talking by anyone in the room.

Do not look at the stopwatch during the test. Instead, mentally count the seconds until the test is finished. For safety and scoring purposes, keep your eyes on the SP at all times, observing them closely throughout the trial. Exact times to failure can be read from the stopwatch after the test is finished. Stop the test after <u>30 seconds</u>, or whenever the subject does something that constitutes a failure (see

Scoring Protocol, page 3-11). Stop the watch, and tell the examinee "OK, you may stop now." <u>Have the examinee step off the foam pad.</u>

Click on the pass or DNP button to record the result, and to record the number of seconds and reason for failure.

If the examinee was able to maintain the stance for 30 seconds, continue with Condition 4.

If the examinee was unable to maintain the stance for 30 seconds, offer to conduct a retrial of the condition by asking, "Can we try that again?" This encourages the SP to do the retrial without sounding optional, or forcing the SP to do a retrial. If necessary, you may allow the subject up to 1 minute to reorient himself between trials. If the examinee agrees to try again, turn the foam pad over. Repeat the condition exactly as before. If the examinee does not want to try again, the balance examination should be terminated (see Section 3.6) by clicking on the "Close" button.

3.3.3.4   Test Condition 4

Turn over the foam pad. Again demonstrating the proper stance (but without standing on the foam), instruct the examinee using the following standard script:

> "This test will be just like the last test; except this time, during the test you will have your eyes closed. When I tell you, close your eyes and stand in the same position—with your feet together and your arms and hands at your waist like this. Remain in this position with your eyes closed for as long as you can or until I ask you to stop. I will let you know when we are ready to begin; and then please do not talk until we are finished with this part of the test. Do you have any questions?"

Direct the examinee to step onto the center of the foam pad, facing the visual target on the door. When the examinee has assumed the correct position, say "Ready? Close your eyes. Start." and begin the timing with the stopwatch. Once the watch is activated, there should be no talking by anyone in the room.

Do not look at the stopwatch during the test. Instead, mentally count the seconds until the test is finished. For safety and scoring purposes, keep your eyes on the SP at all times, observing them closely throughout the trial. Exact times to failure can be read from the stopwatch after the test is finished. Stop the test after <u>30 seconds,</u> or whenever the subject does something which constitutes a failure (see Scoring Protocol below). Stop the watch, and tell the examinee "OK, you may stop now." Have the examinee step off the foam pad.

Record results as mentioned above.

If the examinee was able to maintain the stance for 30 seconds, the balance examination is ended.

If the examinee was unable to maintain the stance for 30 seconds, offer to conduct a retrial of the condition by asking, "Can we try that again?" This encourages the SP to do the retrial without sounding optional, or forcing the SP to do a retrial. If necessary, you may allow the subject up to 1 minute to reorient himself between trials. If the examinee would like to try again, turn over the foam pad. Repeat the condition exactly as before. If the examinee does not want to try again, the balance examination should be terminated.

3.4   Scoring Protocol

Each trial and each condition will be scored as either PASS or DNP (Did not pass). Failure is defined as any occurrence of any of the following within the time interval for a condition (Exhibit 3-5):

■   Movement of the subject's feet from the initial test position (falling, side-stepping, hopping, pivoting, etc.);

■   Movement of the subject's arms off the waist;

■   Eyes open during an eyes-closed condition (i.e., Conditions 2 and 4); or

■   Any intervention by the health technologist to stop the subject from falling.

Increased sway without movement of the feet does not constitute a failure. Talking within the time interval for a condition such that the technologist has to respond to the subject is cause to stop the trial and repeat it, but is not defined as a failure.

In many situations an SP's reactions with the feet, arms, and eyes are nearly simultaneous. In these cases, the health technologist's best judgement must be made with respect to scoring the reason for failure based on vigilant monitoring of the SP.

All trials per condition will be stored in the ISIS database. If the condition is failed, the time to failure (rounded to the nearest second) will also be recorded.

Exhibit 3-5. Choice of reasons for failure of condition

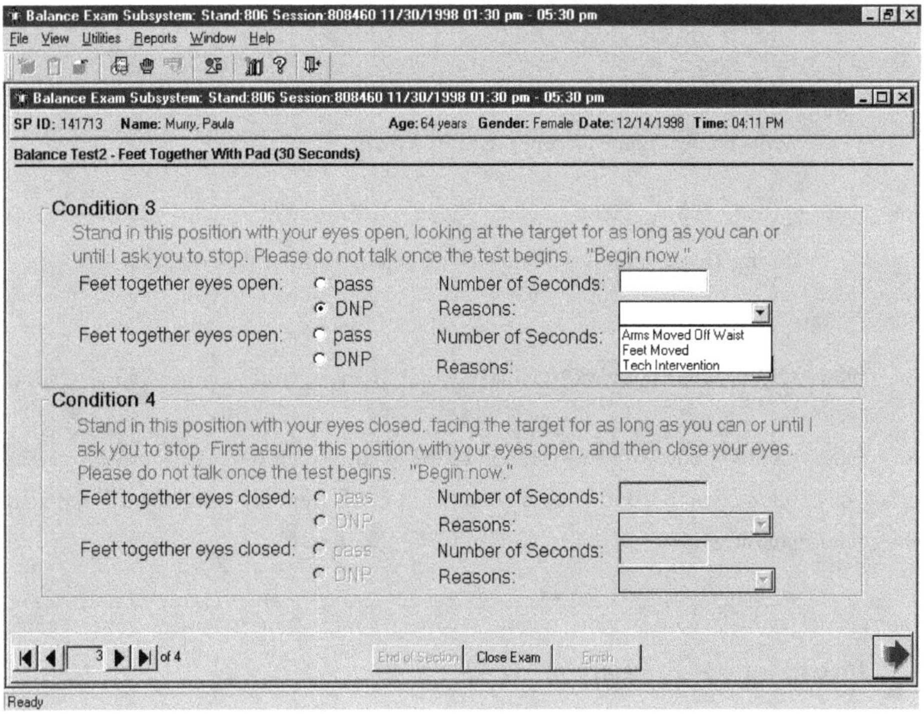

3.5 Safety Protocol

The NHANES balance testing protocol is very simple and straightforward. However, a few precautionary measures are necessary to ensure the safety of examinees who may have trouble with the procedure due to their balance difficulties.

■ Assist the examinee in assuming the test position and in making the transition from one test condition to another, especially when stepping on and off the foam surface.

■ Always stand on a firm surface on the subject's right, with your hands near (but not touching) the grab loop on the safety belt.

■ Ensure that the subject stands close enough to the back wall of the test room that the wall may serve to break a fall if the examinee becomes unstable.

■ Err on the conservative side; even if you are unsure that an examinee is destabilizing or if you are not sure that he or she has recovered balance, grab the loop on the safety belt.

■ Maintain the mind set that the subject could fall at any moment during the test.

While the mentality that an examinee could fall at any time is critical to being ready to prevent a fall, note that the following times during the test pose the greatest risk of destabilization:

- While the examinee is stepping onto the foam and placing his or her feet together;

- While the examinee is stepping off the foam;

- During the first 3 seconds of a new test condition; and

- During Test Conditions 3 and 4 (with greater risk during Condition 4).

3.6 Post-examination Procedures

Each exam will end with presentation of the status screen for your completion. If the exam was a partial, or not done, you need to enter a comment. Logoff from the component is automatic upon completion of the status screen.

3.6.1 Directions to the Examinee

If the examinee inquires about specific results of the balance examination, explain to him or her that you simply conduct the tests and that you are not permitted to interpret any of the results.

Thank the examinee and direct him to the next appropriate station, as prompted by the coordinator on-screen.

3.6.2 Referral

No referrals will be made on the basis of the balance exam. However, the technician can instruct the SP to consult his/her primary care physician if he/she expresses any concern about his/her balance as a result of this test.

4. ADDITIONAL FIELD PROCEDURES

4.1   Start of Stand Procedures

Start of stand procedures for the balance component are simple and straightforward.

First, check that the component's computer hardware and application can be brought up and are in working condition.

Secondly, unpack the equipment necessary for testing: one of the pads, the three belts, and a stopwatch. Place these items on the right side of the shelf below the counter. Place the empty box along with the backup pad, which remains packed, on the left side of the same shelf.

Make sure that the visual target is attached to the back of the door to the room. Attach the instruction card to the side wall of the component room, opposite the wall with the computer, for your reference during examinations.

4.2   Weekly Procedures

At the beginning of each testing week of a stand, unpack the backup foam pad and pack the pad that was used during the previous week. Rotating the foam pads from week to week within a stand helps insure that both remain compliant and usable for testing.

4.3   Care and Maintenance Procedures

The lycra covers of the foam pads require washing at least once per stand. This could be done either at the beginning of the stand, on an off day or half day during the stand, or at the end of the stand. The covers can be machine washed in cold water. If machine dried, a low or no heat setting should be used.

4.4   End of Stand Procedures

The procedures for an end of stand requires only that equipment be packed in the boxes provided and stored securely under the shelf in the component room. All equipment should be accounted for, and any missing items reported immediately to the MEC manager. The inventory of equipment should always match the description provided in Section 2.2.

www.ingramcontent.com/pod-product-compliance
Lightning Source LLC
Chambersburg PA
CBHW081756170526
45167CB00009B/4042